Choose Your Challenge

Designing Personalized Fitness and Nutrition Plans

Table of Contents

Chapter 1. Introduction

In this exclusive Special Report titled 'Choose Your Challenge: Designing Personalized Fitness and Nutrition Plans', we intend to inspire an invigorating journey towards healthy living. Embrace the exhilarating promise of control, clarity, and accomplishment as we delve into the ever-exciting realm of personalized fitness and nutrition. Here's your golden ticket, an opportunity to take charge of your wellness destiny, backed by cohesive plans and strategies that align with your unique physiological needs and lifestyle preferences. So let's traverse this empowering path to physical well-being together, making your health aspirations tangible realities. This report is not just a purchase; it's your ticket to a fulfilling, robust, and vibrant life you always envisioned. Take that rewarding leap towards a healthier you today!

Chapter 2. Understanding the Basics of Nutrition and Fitness

Before making any lifestyle changes, it is crucial to examine the elemental principles that govern our health, especially those related to fitness and nutrition. A deep comprehension of these basics will enlighten you, arming you with the tools necessary to engineer a personalized plan that optimizes your health while remaining cognizant of your individual needs and challenges.

2.1. Defining Nutrition

Nutrition is a scientific discipline that investigates the relationship between dietary intake and our bodies' function. It studies how the substances in the foods we consume promote growth, reproduction, health, and disease prevention.

Our bodies require various nutrients to function correctly, each with specific roles. These include carbohydrates, proteins, fats, vitamins, minerals, fiber, and water. Getting these nutrients in correct proportions is essential for maintaining optimum health.

1. *Carbohydrates* : Primary sources of energy, and include simple carbs like sugar and complex carbs like whole grains and legumes.

2. *Proteins* : Fundamental building blocks of body tissues, proteins also work as enzymes and antibodies. Sources include animal products and plant-based foods like beans and lentils.

3. *Fats* : Essential for brain function, skin health, and absorbing certain vitamins. Healthy fats are found in foods like avocados, oily fish, nuts, and seeds.

4. *Vitamins & Minerals* : Crucial for various bodily functions like immunity, bone health, and energy production, they are present in various foods, including fruits, vegetables, and dairy products.

5. *Fiber* : Promotes a healthy digestive system and can be found in whole grains, fruits, vegetables, and legumes.

6. *Water* : Vital for nearly every process in our body, from temperature regulation to carrying nutrients.

2.2. Nutritional Assessment

Given their crucial roles, understanding your current nutritional status is the starting point for a customized dietary plan. Nutritional assessment can involve various means such as dietary recall and analysis, anthropometric measurements, and lab tests evaluating nutrient levels. This evaluation aids in establishing where changes are needed, offering a roadmap to better nutrition.

2.3. Principles of Balanced Eating

A healthy diet adheres to a balance of nutrients and portion control. Choose diverse foods from each food group, aiming for nutrient-dense options. Portion control is essential - even healthy foods can contribute to weight gain if eaten in excess.

Adopting a diet rich in fruits, vegetables, lean proteins, and whole grains while minimizing ultra-processed foods, saturated fats, and sugars can have a transformative effect on your health, reducing disease risk and promoting vitality.

2.4. Understanding Fitness

Fitness is a state of health and well-being that allows you to perform daily activities with vitality, participate in leisure activities actively, and have a physical readiness to meet unforeseen emergencies. It comprises various components, including cardiovascular endurance, muscular strength and endurance, flexibility, and body composition.

Understanding the different components of fitness is essential because each contributes to a well-rounded fitness routine:

1. *Cardiovascular Endurance* : The efficiency of your heart, lungs, and blood vessels to deliver oxygen to your body during prolonged exercise.

2. *Muscular Strength* : The maximum amount of force that a muscle can exert against some form of resistance in a single effort.

3. *Muscular Endurance* : The ability of a muscle to lift weight or perform repetitive movements over a prolonged period.

4. *Flexibility* : The ability to move your joints through a full range of motion without discomfort or injury.

5. *Body Composition* : The relative amounts of muscle, bone, water, and fat in the body, impacting overall fitness and health.

Achieving a balance between these components not only boosts your overall fitness levels but also reduces the risks of injury and enhances your quality of life.

2.5. Importance of Fitness Assessment

Just as with nutrition, a detailed fitness assessment is your starting point when aiming to improve your fitness levels. This involves gauging your cardiovascular fitness, strength, flexibility, and understanding your body composition. Such assessments provide a precise starting point and help design a personalized fitness plan congruent with your abilities and goals.

2.6. Principles of Exercise

The American College of Sports Medicine recommends a mix of aerobic exercises, resistance training, flexibility exercises, and balance exercises for most adults. Begin with light to moderate intensity activities and gradually increase intensity as your fitness improves. Remember to warm up before and cool down after your workouts to prepare the body and assist in recovery, respectively.

A personalized fitness plan respects your current fitness level, goals, available time, and likes or dislikes. Keep variety in your routine to avoid boredom and to challenge different muscle groups. And most importantly, prioritize consistency over perfection.

Achieving a balanced lifestyle that encompasses both optimal nutrition and suited fitness practices is not a one-time act but a continuous journey. Empowered with the understanding of the basic principles of nutrition and fitness, you will now be able to lay solid foundations for your personalized health journey that are both sustainable and enjoyable.

Chapter 3. Assessing Your Personal Health and Fitness Level

To start the journey towards a healthier lifestyle, it's crucial to get a baseline assessment of your current health and fitness levels.

3.1. Initial Insight

Understanding where we're starting allows us to visualize our goals better, comprehend the journey that lies ahead, and customize the fitness and nutrition plans to best suit our needs. Taking assessments gives us concrete, quantifiable data about our health, fitness, and nutritional status, which is arguably the most critical step on the journey to wellness.

3.2. Background Health Check

The first essential goal is to evaluate our background health status. This means exploring our past and present medical histories, allergies, significant illnesses, surgeries, and medications. It also includes our family's medical history, which can provide clues to potential hereditary health issues. Comprehensive medical assessments will give us holistic insight about our physical health condition and needs, and they are vital while designing a captivating personal fitness and nutrition plan.

3.3. Self-Health Perception

Another crucial component is our self-perception of health. It's about how we assess our own health—both physical and mental. For instance, ranking physical health on a scale from 1-10 may differ vastly from person to person, based on their personal experiences and understanding of health. Similarly, keeping an eye on mental health is essential as stress, anxiety, and depression can gravely affect our physiological well-being.

3.4. Nutritional Assessment

A nutritional assessment is next on the agenda. This evaluation consists of keeping track of what we consume, how frequently, and in what quantities. Doing so helps identify trends and discrepancies in our dietary habits that can affect our health. Using tools like a food diary or health apps helps systematically record and analyze this. Additionally, testing for nutrient levels can detect deficiencies or excesses that need immediate attention.

3.5. Fitness Assessment

The fitness level assessment provides tangible metrics about our physical state. This can be initiated with basic fitness tests like cardiovascular endurance tests (e.g., 1 mile walk or run), strength tests (like push-ups or sit-ups), flexibility tests (like sit and reach), and body composition tests (body mass index or BMI, body fat percentage). The results from these evaluations give us tangible benchmarks against which we can measure our progress.

3.6. Sleep Evaluation

A worthwhile evaluation is assessing our sleep patterns. Sleep is often overlooked but plays a pivotal role in our physiological health. Quality and quantity of sleep impact our recovery, energy levels, mood, and even food cravings. Therefore, analyzing our sleep patterns, troubleshooting sleep disturbances, and ensuring we get the optimal amount of sleep each night can have a transformative effect on our overall health and wellness journey.

3.7. Stress Influences

Assessing stress levels is also important. Prolonged high-stress levels can lead to a host of health issues including heart disease, weight gain, sleep problems, and a weakened immune system. Recognizing our stressors and developing coping mechanisms usually aids in mitigating the negative impacts of stress on our health. Techniques such as meditation, yoga, or even basic deep breathing exercises can all help in managing stress levels.

3.8. Habits and Lifestyle Examination

Lastly, our habits and lifestyle choices play a substantial role in defining our health and fitness. Habits such as smoking, alcohol consumption, drug use, and even sitting for extended periods can significantly impact health and longevity. Acknowledging these habits and working towards reducing or eliminating them can induce considerable positive shifts in our health and wellbeing.

In summary, developing an in-depth understanding of your current health and fitness level forms the foundation of personalized fitness and nutrition plans. This crucial initial assessment enables us to highlight areas of focus, set achievable goals, and embark on a healthier lifestyle journey attuned to our unique personal needs and preferences. It's essential to honor this process, trust it, and let it guide us towards becoming the best version of ourselves. Remember, health is an ongoing journey, not a destination. Be patient with yourself, celebrate your small victories, and never lose sight of why you started.

Chapter 4. Setting Attainable Fitness Goals

The inclination to set fitness goals arises from the firm resolve to transform one's health for the better. There is an exhilarating promise in the vision of your fitter, healthier self. However, the journey to this vision requires strategic planning - a map that charts your course, each step demarcated with precision and prudence. Let's embark on that journey together.

4.1. Understanding Fitness Goals and Their Importance

Fitness goals form the nucleus of your fitness journey. A clear, achievable fitness objective offers you a tangible target, helping streamline your workout routines and diet plans. It provides the motivation needed to break through the toughest barriers on your health and wellness journey, pushing you to go that extra yard when the going gets tough.

Fitness goals also provide a measure of your progress. You know you are moving in the right direction when you see yourself inch closer towards your goals with each passing week. Having achievable goals allows for timely revisions and adjustments based on your performance, preventing stagnation and ensuring continued progress.

Finally, fitness goals imbibe the culture of discipline and consistency within you. They help foster a better relationship with your body, teaching you to listen to, understand, and respect the signals it sends.

4.2. Setting S.M.A.R.T. Fitness Goals

Perhaps the most effective way to set fitness goals is by adhering to the S.M.A.R.T. principle. S.M.A.R.T. stands for Specific, Measurable, Achievable, Relevant, and Time-Bound.

Table 1. A S.M.A.R.T. Fitness Goal Explained

S (Specific)	**Your goal should be clear and specific. Instead of saying, "I want to lose weight", say, "I want to lose 10 pounds."**
M (Measurable)	Your goal should be quantifiable. Numbers help in accurately gauging your progress.
A (Achievable)	Make sure the goal you set is reasonable and within your physical capabilities to prevent burnouts.
R (Relevant)	Your goal should be in line with your broader wellness objectives,
T (Time-bound)	Assign a timeline to your goal to ensure disciplined pursuit.

4.3. Creating a Customized Workout Plan to Achieve Your Goals

To translate your fitness goals into realities, a personalized workout plan is critical. As no two individuals are the same, neither should their fitness plans be.

When devising a workout plan, the cardinal rule of thumb is to consider factors such as age, current health status, lifestyle habits, and physical limitations, if any. Remember to gradually scale intensity levels, especially if you are new to exercising or returning after a hiatus.

Your fitness goals also dictate the type of workout you should pursue. If your goal is to build muscle, include more strength training exercises in your regime. On the other hand, if your goal is weight loss, a combination of high-intensity interval training (HIIT) and cardio exercises could work best.

Remember, exercise is not just about losing weight or building muscle. It also enhances mental well-being, improves body function, and increases longevity. So, aim to build a regimen that cultivates comprehensive fitness.

4.4. Adapting Nutrition to Facilitate Fitness Goals

Physical exercise alone may not fetch you your desired results. Your nutrition plays an equally important role in achieving your fitness goals. Understanding this correlation is paramount when planning meals.

If your goal is weight loss, focus on creating a calorie deficit through a balanced diet that's nutrient-dense but low in calories. If muscle-building is your goal, ensure you're getting ample protein to aid muscle recovery and growth.

Tailoring meals according to workout schedules can also elevate performance and recovery. For instance, consuming easily digestible carbohydrates and proteins before a workout can provide fuel, while the same post-workout aids recovery.

4.5. Tracking and Evaluating Progress

It's important to track your progress along the journey to your fitness goals. Regular monitoring will help you adjust your strategies as per the results. This could be as simple as keeping a workout journal or using digital fitness apps to track your workouts, nutrition, and performance.

Remember, progress plateaus are natural. Rather than get disheartened, see them as opportunities for revision and recalibration of your strategies. You may need to make tweaks to your workout or nutrition, or sometimes, even your goals.

4.6. Embracing Patience and Persistence

The journey to fitness is not an overnight sprint but a marathon that demands patience and persistence. Goals may take longer to reach than expected, mudding paths with frustration. It's vital to remain resilient during these testing times, recollecting your reasons for setting out on this journey and all the progress you have made since.

As an often-understated principle, remember the 'two-day rule' – never skip your workout two days in a row. The occasional day of rest is beneficial, but breaking the momentum regularly can derail progress. In the end, consistent daily efforts, however small, outweigh sporadic, highly intensive ones.

In conclusion, setting attainable fitness goals is a masterstroke that can invigorate your journey towards better health and wellness. Coupled with a personalized plan reflecting your lifestyle and capabilities, these goals not only promise physical transformation but also impart valuable life skills such as discipline, patience, and resilience. So set your S.M.A.R.T. goal today and stride confidently on your path to holistic fitness.

Chapter 5. Crafting a Personalized Nutrition Blueprint

Introduction to Personalized Nutrition

Paving the way towards a healthier life involves a holistic approach. This means understanding that our dietary needs are as unique as our fingerprints. Personalized nutrition recognizes these unique characteristics, offering a customized approach to nourishing our bodies. An effective nutrition plan takes into account individual genetic, phenotypic and behavioral characteristics, carving an exclusive wellness path for us.

5.1. The Importance of Personalized Nutrition

The concept of 'one size fits all' is defunct in the arena of nutrition. A diet plan suited for one may not fit another due to the complex interplay between genetics, lifestyle, and personal health goals. Personalized nutrition plans are developed with a comprehensive understanding of an individual's unique needs to ensure optimal health and wellness. They play a significant role in preventative healthcare, maintaining body weight, enhancing athletic performance, and managing chronic illnesses.

5.2. Discovering Your Unique Nutritional Needs

Drawing your body's nutritional blueprint requires taking into consideration an array of factors. These include your age, gender, weight, height, body composition, physical activity level, basal metabolic rate (BMR), and any pre-existing health conditions.

Another factor is genetic predisposition. Genetic analysis provides insights about how your body metabolizes nutrients from the food you consume. It can shed light on your susceptibility to obesity, type 2 diabetes, and how your body responds to different types of diets.

Food preferences are another aspect affecting your diet blueprint. Personal food choices, influenced by culture, habits, and palates, are crucial in designing an appealing and sustainable nutrition plan.

5.3. Establishing Balanced Dietary Guidelines

After discovering your unique dietary needs, it becomes imperative to sketch balanced dietary guidelines. A balanced diet is an assembly of foods from all food groups in adequate proportions to fuel bodily functions efficiently. It is key to include macro and micronutrients, such as proteins, carbohydrates, fat, vitamins, and minerals in your meal plan.

Macro and micronutrient distribution should align with your unique requirements. For instance, a physically active person may require a higher proportion of protein and complex carbohydrates, whereas someone with a sedentary lifestyle could benefit from moderate protein, low carbohydrates and higher fiber intake.

5.4. The Art of Meal Planning

Once dietary guidelines have been established, we can step into the practice of meal planning. Meal planning ensures the smooth execution of your diet blueprint. It involves developing menus based on preferred meal frequencies - could be 3 meals a day or 5 smaller portions.

For better compliance, it's essential that the meals planned are diverse yet conforming to the dietary guidelines. Meal planning can also consider the cultural, ethical, and personal preferences to ensure the plan remains enjoyable for maximum adherence.

5.5. Making Room for Time and Convenience

An often overlooked, but important aspect of personalized nutrition is understanding the individual's available time and convenience for meal preparation. Ready-to-eat options or easy recipes could come to the rescue of those short on time.

5.6. Incorporating Mindful Eating

Mindful eating practices can be implemented to help one reconnect with their body's hunger and satiety cues, encouraging a healthier relationship with food. It nurtures your physical health and aids psychological well-being, reinforcing a holistic culmination to the nutritional blueprint.

5.7. Continuous Evaluation and Adjustments

Finally, it's essential to evaluate the effectiveness of the plan by tracking changes in body composition, energy levels, performance, and mood. The nutritional blueprint is a dynamic document that requires periodic refreshment and adjustment based on these metrics.

In conclusion, developing a personalized nutritional blueprint is a meticulous process that requires an understanding of various biomarkers, lifestyle habits, and personal preferences. Working with a professional nutritionist, you can have a blueprint that's custom-made, keeping your unique dietary needs and preferences in mind. This sets the stage for healthier eating habits, paving the way towards achieving your optimal health and wellness goals.

Remember, your nutritional plan is a powerful tool in creating the fulfilling, robust, and vibrant life you always envisioned. Here's to making healthier choices, one meal at a time.

Chapter 6. Designing a Customized Exercise Plan

We begin by understanding that your exercise regimen should align with both your fitness goals and your individual body composition. There is no one-size-fits-all approach; understanding your needs is critically important.

6.1. Understanding Your Body Type

Knowing your body composition is an essential first step to designing a personalized exercise plan. Not all bodies are built the same way, and different types gain and lose weight differently. In the 1940s, psychologist William Herbert Sheldon classified bodies into three categories: ectomorphs (lean and long, with difficulty building muscle), mesomorphs (muscular and well-built, with a high metabolism and responsive muscle cells), and endomorphs (high body fat, often pear-shaped, with a tendency to store fat).

Identifying your body type helps to tailor your exercise program to your specific needs. For instance, if you're an endomorph, you might fare better on a regimen centred around cardio to help burn off extra fat. Suppose you're an ectomorph, weight training might be more suited to help build muscle mass.

6.2. Setting Fitness Goals

Your personalised exercise plan will be heavily influenced by what you hope to achieve. If you're on a weight loss journey, your program might focus more on high-intensity cardio. Muscle gain would entail a heavier emphasis on strength training. It's important to quantify your goals; for example, aim to lose 10 pounds or aim to bench press 200 pounds. This specificity makes your steps towards your goal measurable and thus more manageable.

6.3. Balancing Cardio and Strength Training

A comprehensive exercise plan includes both cardio and strength training, regardless of your fitness goals. Cardiovascular activities like running, cycling, or swimming boost your heart health, help to reduce blood pressure, and aid in weight loss. On the other hand, strength training activities such as weight lifting or resistance workouts help you build muscle, boost metabolism, and increase bone density. Striking a balance between the two ensures overall fitness. An ideal proportion would be 150 minutes per week of moderate aerobic activity plus two days of strength training exercises.

6.4. Creating an Exercise Schedule

Mark your calendar with specific tasks for each day of the week - Monday for swimming, Tuesday for strength training, so on and so forth. Adhering to this schedule will ensure consistency, which in turn will lead to significant fitness improvements over time. Also, always allot some time for a proper warm-up before any intense workout and a cool down afterwards to prevent injuries and speed up recovery.

6.5. Tracking Your Progress

Having a fitness journal to keep track of your workouts is an effective way to measure progress. Document your activities, the duration, the intensity, and your feelings post-workout. This provides you a concrete record of your progress, showing you how much you've improved over time.

6.6. Taking Rest Days

Rest is just as important as your workouts. Remember to incorporate rest days in your schedule to allow your body to recover and build muscle. Over-exercising might lead to fatigue, injuries, and a decrease in motivation.

6.7. Hiring a Professional

If you're new to exercising and feeling a bit lost, hiring a personal trainer can be beneficial. A professional will provide guidance, ensure you're doing exercises correctly to prevent injury, and keep you motivated.

In conclusion, designing a customized exercise plan necessitates understanding your body type, setting clear fitness goals, balancing cardio and strength activities, creating a well-defined schedule, tracking progress, incorporating rest days and potentially hiring a professional. It's a beautiful voyage towards a healthier you, and every step you take is progress. So begin today and embrace the exhilaration of this journey.

Remember, it's not about perfection; it's about progress. You don't need to be the fastest, the strongest, or the fittest; you just need to be better than you were yesterday. You are your only competition, so strive to out-do yourself every day. Success in fitness, like any other area of life, is about taking small, consistent steps towards your goal. Onward, towards a healthier, happier you.

Chapter 7. Mastering Portion Control and Meal Timing

Portion control and meal timing are two crucial aspects of a personalized fitness and nutrition plan. Not only are they key to maintaining a healthy weight, but they also play a significant role in our bodies' metabolic processes. Understanding the importance of portion control and meal timing and incorporating them in your daily routine can lead you towards a healthier and more balanced lifestyle.

7.1. The Importance of Portion Control

Portion control is about understanding how much of each type of food you should eat to maintain a balanced and healthy diet. Over the years, portion sizes have been gradually increasing in restaurants and at home leading to an overconsumption of calories. Studies show this is a significant factor contributing to the rise in obesity rates.

Knowing the right portion sizes can help you balance your diet. When you control your portions, you limit your intake of unhealthy foods, but you also ensure you are getting enough nutrients from all food groups. A balanced diet that includes the right portions of each food group can provide you with the necessary vitamins, minerals, and other nutrients your body needs to be healthy.

It's important to understand serving sizes and how they compare to the portion sizes you eat. Serving sizes are standardized measurements of foods and help you understand nutritional information, while portion size is the amount you choose to eat. For instance, while a serving of pasta on a food label might be 1/2 cup, you might choose to eat a 1 cup portion at home.

You might be wondering what a portion size looks like. Typically, a portion of protein such as beef, chicken, or fish should be about the size of your palm. A serving of carbohydrates, like bread or pasta, should be about the size of your fist. And a serving of fat, such as butter or oil, should be about the size of your thumb. By scaling your meals in this way, you can help ensure that you're getting a balanced diet.

7.2. Mindful Eating and Portion Control

Mindful eating is a way to help you control your portions. Instead of eating mindlessly and possibly overeating, when you practice mindful eating you take the time to savor your food. You pay attention to your hunger and fullness cues, and you are more aware of how much you are eating.

Start by serving yourself smaller portions. If you find that you're still hungry after finishing your meal, you can add more food. This can help you avoid eating larger portions simply because they are in front of you. Make sure to eat without distractions, like TV or smartphones, to pay full attention to your meals.

Being aware of why you eat can also help with portion control. Are you actually hungry, or are you bored, fatigued or stressed? Understanding these patterns can help you avoid eating when you're not really hungry and choose more appropriate responses to your feelings.

7.3. The Art of Meal Timing

Meal timing is the practice of eating meals and snacks at specific times throughout the day to optimize health. It's based on the idea that syncing your eating patterns with your body's natural rhythms can improve your metabolism, digestion, and overall health.

Eating at regular intervals helps your body regulate its metabolism —
it knows when it can expect food and it learns to optimally process
and use the energy from that food. Plus, regular eating times can
prevent overeating or under-eating, both of which can have negative
impacts on your health.

Three meals a day is a common pattern of meal timing for many
people. However, some people may prefer to eat smaller meals more
often. Eating five or six smaller meals throughout the day can help
keep your metabolism active and can prevent overeating by keeping
your hunger at bay.

Another concept that has gained popularity is time-restricted eating
or intermittent fasting. This concept includes a defined "eating
window," such as from 10 a.m. to 6 p.m., which is believed to align
better with our bodies' natural circadian rhythms. This can lead to
better digestion, improvement in sleep, and potential weight loss.
However, it's important to follow these protocols under the guidance
of a healthcare professional.

7.4. Syncing Your Eating Habits with Your Lifestyle

Your lifestyle and routine can greatly influence your meal timing. If
you're an early riser, you might benefit from an earlier breakfast to
kickstart your metabolism for the day. On the other hand, if you tend
to be more active in the evening, you might prefer a larger lunch and
a lighter dinner.

For those who exercise regularly, nutrient timing can be an
important consideration. Aiming for a balanced intake of protein and
carbohydrates before and after a workout can maximize
performance and recovery. For example, eating a small snack of

banana and almond butter 1-2 hours before workout provides energy and then having a protein-rich meal after the workout helps with recovery.

In conclusion, mastering portion control and meal timing is a reliable step in the direction of personal health and fitness. It allows you to connect deeper with your body's intrinsic needs and reactions to different food groups and eating patterns. By adopting these practices, you can enjoy a more balanced, energetic, and healthier lifestyle.

Chapter 8. Countering Common Fitness and Nutrition Myths

Navigating the sphere of fitness and nutrition can often prove to be quite challenging, largely due to the proliferation of numerous well-intentioned but misleading myths. Often touted as truths, these myths can create confusion, and in worst-case scenarios, jeopardize our health. The mission of this chapter, therefore, is to debunk these common myths, and arm you with the correct, science-back information you need to kick-start your journey to wellness and maintain a healthy lifestyle.

8.1. Deconstructing Myth 1: Crash Diets lead to Permanent Weight Loss

Many often subscribe to crash diets in hopes of rapid weight loss. The allure is potent: quick results with minimal time. However, a key aspect to understand is that these diets are essentially starvation regimes that might lead to temporary weight loss but result in longer-term harm.

Crash diets often drastically squeeze calorie intake, forcing the body into a 'starvation mode.' While this induces quick weight loss, it comprises mainly water loss and muscle mass reduction. The moment your body reverts to normal eating patterns, it begins storing calories, leading to an eventual increase in weight. Worse, it may lead to serious mental and physical health issues such as eating disorders, malnutrition, and other conditions.

8.2. Tackling Myth 2: All Fats are Bad

For years, fat has been the villainized element in our diets, responsible for weight gain, high cholesterol levels and various health issues. However, the reality is far from this blanket stereotype. In fact, our bodies need fat – the right kind of fat.

There are two main types of fat: unsaturated and saturated. Unsaturated fats, found in foods like avocados, olive oil, and salmon, are beneficial. They can help decrease bad cholesterol levels, reduce the risk of heart disease, and provide essential fatty acids.

On the other hand, while saturated fats – found in full-fat dairy, pork, beef – consumed in excess, can raise bad cholesterol levels and risk of cardiovascular diseases. So instead of eliminating all fats, aim for a balanced diet of essential fats.

8.3. Demystifying Myth 3: You Must Detox Your Body with Juice Cleanses

The idea of 'detoxing' and 'cleansing' the body with a strict regimen of juices and smoothies has gained considerable popularity recently. Unfortunately, this is a misguided concept.

Our bodies are sublimely equipped to flush out toxins through the liver, kidneys, and digestive system, needing no exclusive juice diet for detoxification. Moreover, these juices are typically high in sugar and low in protein, leading to energy spikes and crashes. They also don't have enough fiber, a nutrient crucial for digestion and feeling full.

8.4. Disputing Myth 4: More Exercise Means More Weight Loss

While burning more calories does contribute to weight loss, this equation isn't as simple as it seems. As you increase the intensity or duration of your workouts, your body's energy needs increase. This can make you feel hungrier and consume more calories than you burned, limiting the total weight loss.

Furthermore, excessive exercise without balanced nutrition and recovery periods can lead to injuries or other health complications. It's about finding the right balance and ensuring your workout routine fits your nutritional intake.

8.5. Unveiling Myth 5: Skipping Meals Can Help Lose Weight

Another harmful myth is the idea of skipping meals to shed pounds. In reality, this practice can lead to the opposite effect. When you skip a meal, your body shifts into starvation mode, slowing metabolism and conserving energy.

Skipping meals also often leads to overeating during the next meal, negating any calories that may have been saved. Instead of skipping, opt for balanced, nutritious meals that fuel your body's daily activities healthily.

8.6. Challenging Myth 6: Carbs are the Enemy

Carbohydrates have been unjustly villainized, but not all carbs are bad. Many foods high in complex carbs, like whole grains, fruits, and legumes, provide necessary nutrients and dietary fiber, helping control weight and lower the risk of heart disease.

The real enemy are the simple carbs found in processed foods and drinks, which have been stripped of their fiber and nutrients, leaving behind essentially empty calories.

In conclusion, many common fitness and nutrition myths can cloud our understanding of healthy practices. It's crucial to be well-informed about the realities of these myths as we navigate our way to a healthier lifestyle. This knowledge can dispel the confusion, helping us make healthier choices and enjoy a balanced and fulfilling journey of fitness and nutrition.

Chapter 9. The Role of Motivation and Persuasion in Fitness Success

The aspiration to achieve optimal health is universal, yet the steps towards this destination may stand shrouded in enormous challenges. As we delve into the crux of fostering healthy habits, it's imperative to underscore two keystone elements of the journey: motivation and persuasion. These dynamic forces pave the way, transforming the overwhelming roadmap into a worthwhile journey of self-discovery and self-celebration. Harnessing these elements to propel towards fitness goals can anticipate success, making the process of transformation far enjoyable and rewarding.

9.1. Understanding Motivation and Persuasion

Motivation is your internal drive, the fuel propelling you to take actions. It can be intrinsic, driven by personal gratification, or extrinsic, influenced by external rewards. On the other hand, persuasion taps into the cognitive, emotional, and social aspects, encouraging a behavior change. Essentially, motivation initiates the change while persuasion shapes and sustains it, ensuring the transition from intent to action to habit edification.

In the context of fitness, motivation pushes you towards the starting line while persuasion guarantees you continue with the regimen even when the initial adrenaline rush dissipates. The fitness journey often starts with a spark of motivation—an emerging health concern, a sudden realization, or a goal weight. However, lasting change requires the power of persuasion—convincing oneself of the immeasurable benefits, both immediate and long term. A persuasive mind, coupled with strong motivation, can tackle the most exhausting workout circuits or the strictest dietary plan.

9.2. Explore Your Motivation Source

Before embarking on your fitness journey, it's crucial to identify your unique motivation types. Understanding your specific triggers can ensure you maintain that impetus throughout your journey. This self-exploration can reveal intrinsic motivators (like the joy of a good workout) and extrinsic motivators (like reaching your target weight). Once identified, fueling these motivators can optimize your chances of not just meeting but surpassing fitness milestones.

9.3. Fostering Sustainable Motivation

In the fitness world, there's a phrase "Motivation gets you started, habit keeps you going." Hence, while motivation acts as a catalyst, the challenge lies in maintaining that level of enthusiasm. Here are a few strategies to keep your motivation engine ignited:

- Set specific, achievable and measurable goals. Start with smaller goals and gradually increase the stakes. Every accomplished goal will fuel renewed motivation.

- Track your progress. A visual representation of your fitness journey can serve as a motivational boost.

- Share your plans and achievements with others. The culture of celebration can act as motivators.

- Try group exercises, fitness challenges, or hire a personal trainer. These extrinsic factors can enhance your fitness motivation.

9.4. Strategies for Persuasion in Fitness

Persuasion in fitness involves persuading oneself of the need and benefits of a consistently healthy lifestyle. Persuasive messages can come from external sources, such as a health coach or personal trainer, but the most powerful persuasion is self-persuasion. Consider these strategies for self-persuasion:

- Associate positive emotions with your fitness routine.

- Extrapolate the immediate benefits to translate to long term ones.

- Frame fitness goals as an extension to your self-identity.

9.5. Motivation and Persuasion: An Intrinsic Symbiosis

We've dissected motivation and persuasion separately, yet their true power lies in their collaborative function. Motivation surges from deep within, serves as your launching pad, and fuels your journey. Simultaneously, persuasion, internal or external, unveils the 'why' behind your actions, provides a continuous nudge, reinforcing belief in the endeavor's worth, and transforms motivation into a habit.

The symbiosis of motivation and persuasion sets the tone for a successful fitness journey. By fostering motivation and leveraging persuasion, a daunting fitness journey can morph into an engaging practice of self-improvement, underlining the positive correlation between physical health and mental wellbeing.

In conclusion, while the customization of fitness and nutrition plans plays a key role in health management, the crucial unaddressed variable is the individual's mindset. A paradigm shift towards an empowered mindset harnessed by motivation and persuasion does not only secure success in the fitness realm but also transcends to other life aspects, spotlighting the all-encompassing nature of these dynamic forces.

Remember, the journey of a thousand miles begins with a single step; allow motivation to ignite that step and persuasion to ensure each following stride is one closer to your fitness finish line.

Chapter 10. Comfortably Integrating Changes into Your Lifestyle

Starting a new journey towards a healthier lifestyle can seem daunting. But knowing how to gradually incorporate it into your daily routine without discomfort, stress or upheaval is a game-changer. And that's precisely what we're going to discover together.

Let's start with how you can successfully locate and make those productive changes, then allow them to blossom and evolve into beneficial habits for lifelong well-being.

10.1. Understanding the Status Quo: Starting Where You Are

An essential first step towards lasting lifestyle change is understanding your current habits and behaviors. Spend some time observing your daily patterns and noting the things that you do regularly. These could be everyday activities like having a morning cup of coffee, taking a lunchbreak at a specific time, watching tv in the evening, or going for a late-night snack. Collectively, these habits define your status quo and provide the framework within which new, healthier habits can be implemented.

10.2. Setting SMART Goals: The Bedrock of Change

Once you are familiar with your current lifestyle patterns, it's time to set clear, attainable targets for the changes you want to make. One effective method is to create SMART goals—Specific, Measurable, Achievable, Relevant, and Time-bound.

Specific: Be precise about the change you wish to make. Instead of setting a vague goal like "exercise more", specify what kind of exercise, how often, and for how long. This might look like: "Go for a thirty-minute run three times a week."

Measurable: Make sure that you can track your progress. If your goal is to increase fruit and vegetable intake, you might measure this by aiming to "eat five servings of fruits and vegetables every day."

Achievable: Ensure your goal is realistic and achievable for you. If you've never run before, aiming to run a marathon in a month isn't realistic. Scale it back and set achievable targets like "jogging for 10 minutes each day."

Relevant: Ensure your goal aligns with your broader health and wellness objectives. If your larger goal is to decrease stress levels, then an appropriate goal may be "practicing mindfulness meditation for 15 minutes in the morning."

Time-bound: Provide a timeframe for your goal to keep you focused and motivated. An example may be "losing 5kg in three months."

10.3. Gradual Integrations: Small Steps for Big Wins

Rather than making drastic changes all at once, gradually introduce new habits. For instance, if your goal is to run for 30 minutes daily, you could start by incorporating ten minutes of running into your routine, incrementally increasing the duration. Or if your target is to consume five servings of fruits and vegetables a day, you can start by adding one serving at a time.

10.4. Integrating Physical Activity

Regular physical activity is vital for health and well-being. It can be anything that gets your body moving and increases your heart rate. Here are a few ways you can incorporate more physical activity into your everyday life:

- Try to find activities that you enjoy. If you love nature, consider hiking or biking outdoors. If you enjoy dancing, consider taking a local dance class or use online dance workout videos.

- Where possible, walk or cycle instead of driving or using public transport. This method is not just good for your health, but also beneficial for the environment.

- Incorporate exercise into your daily activities. For instance, do a few push-ups while waiting for your coffee to brew or take a brisk walk during your lunch break.

- Make exercise a social activity. Invite a friend to join you for a morning jog or meet for a workout session. It can make the activity more enjoyable and increase your chances of sticking with it.

10.5. Integrating Healthy Eating Habits

Equally, constantly determining what to eat takes its toll. Here's how you can seamlessly integrate healthy eating habits into your lifestyle:

- Meal planning and meal prepping can be incredibly helpful. Allocate one day a week to plan your meals, go grocery shopping, and prep some meals in advance. You could cook large portions and separate them into individual containers.

- Aim for a balanced plate at every meal: half the plate filled with veggies, a quarter with lean protein, and a quarter with complex carbohydrates.

- Educate yourself about nutrition so that you can make informed choices about what you eat.

- Stay hydrated. Often, the body can mistake dehydration for hunger. Aim to drink at least 8 glasses of water a day.

10.6. The Role of Consistency and Patience

Finally, remember that change doesn't happen overnight. Many people give up because they don't see immediate results. Persistence and gradual improvement are what lead to big changes. Also, keep in mind that minor slip-ups are a normal part of making lifestyle changes. Don't let them discourage you. Instead, learn from them and keep going.

By understanding your current habits, setting SMART goals, and gradually introducing new ones, you'll be better equipped to integrate lasting changes into your lifestyle comfortably. It may take time, but with patience and consistency, these healthier lifestyle habits will become second nature. Remember, it's not about perfection; it's about continual progress towards a healthier, happier you.

Chapter 11. Progress Tracking and Ongoing Adaptations

One of the foundational stones to a solid and effective personalized fitness and nutrition plan is the tracking of progress and making ongoing adaptations. The importance of these elements cannot be overstated. It's essentially about understanding that health and wellness is a journey, not a destination.

11.1. Understanding the Importance of Progress Tracking

Your journey towards fitness and nutrition is a dynamic process that will evolve with time. One of the chief tools that will offer you a roadmap to navigate this ever-shifting terrain is progress tracking.

Progress tracking is a necessary tool in achieving your goals, offering critical insights into your success, identifying potential inefficiencies, and directing changes. It's all about data. Accurate, relevant, and meaningful data provide the information necessary to make informed decisions about your health. It provides a clear picture of your current state of health and fitness, illuminating the path towards your ultimate goals.

There are numerous ways you can track your progress, each with its own set of benefits and complexities. From subjective assessments like perceiving an increase in energy, mood upliftment or better fitting clothes, to the objective metrics of body composition scans, routine blood tests, or performance records, progress tracking can vary greatly according to personal preferences, resources, and needs.

11.2. Embracing The Art of Ongoing Adaptations

Ease and familiarity can sometimes be the enemy of progress. Our bodies, incredibly adaptive machines that they are, eventually learn to work efficiently (with less energy expenditure) on familiar workout routines or dietary patterns. When this plateau arrives, it's time to recalibrate your fitness and nutrition strategy with ongoing adaptations.

Adaptations involve tweaking, substitifying, or diversifying routines, essentially introducing novelty to keep your body challenged. This could come in several forms: A shift from high-intensity workouts to more resistance training, altering macronutrient ratios, timing of meal or trying a new sport or activity.

The process of adaptations is not driven by plateau alone. It caters to the broader spectrum of life's transitions: age, lifestyle changes, health status shifts, change in goals and more.

11.3. How to Monitor Your Progress Efficiently

Start with defining clear, specific, measurable and realistic goals. Identify the metrics that define these goals: for instance, if your goal is weight loss, tracking body weight becomes one of the crucial metrics.

Next, choose suitable tracking tools. Possibilities are endless here: nutrition tracking apps, high-tech fitness trackers, routine blood tests, dietary records, workout logs or wellness journals. The key is to choose tools that are accessible, reliable, and convenient.

Regular and consistent tracking are the essence of effective progress monitoring. Be it daily, weekly, or monthly, establishing a routine and sticking to it is crucial. Regularity dishes out a comprehensive databank to work on, capturing various subtle nuances that random tracking might miss.

Always remember, the tracked data needs to be evaluated in the right context. It's crucial to understand that weight, BMI, or calorie count are not the sole determinants of your health status. Subjective experiences and adaption to synergy between different measurements is as essential as the hard numbers.

11.4. Facilitating Effective Adaptations

Adaptations should be rational, equitable and gradual. Firstly, identify the area requiring adjustment. This could be an extended workout plateau, a deficiency highlighted by a blood test, or simply a feeling of boredom from routine.

Next, brainstorm and plan possible adjustments. It could include trying new workout forms, experimenting with different workout intensities, adjusting meal sizes, altering nutrient compositions or experimenting with meal timings.

Lastly, implement and track. Ensure the changes don't disrupt your routine drastically, and be patient to allow results to show. You can then adjust as required, making sure the plan remains sustainable, enjoyable and in sync with your goals.

Remember, no matter how small an adaptation seems, it can have significant impacts on your overall fitness and nutrition journey. So, yield to the power of small, gradual changes and let your body adapt and respond.

11.5. Conclusion: The Power of Progress Tracking and Ongoing Adaptations

The route towards a healthier and more fulfilling lifestyle can sometimes seem complicated. But equipped with the right tools and strategies, you can navigate with relative ease and confidence. Your commitment to monitor your progress and making relevant modifications is a testament to your desire to improve. It puts you in the driver's seat for steering through your health expedition, ultimately propelling you towards your goals.

Your health journey is uniquely yours. Therefore, customize your strategies, listen to your body, and enjoy the ride. After all, progress in fitness and nutrition is about enhancing the quality of life, not just about the destination! Remember, regular progress tracking and making ongoing adaptations mark the difference between a health chasing and a health thriving individual. Here's to you joining the latter!